AFFIRMATIONS FOR PREGNANT WOMEN

500 Uplifting Mantras for Expectant Mothers

Jordan Parry

Copyright © 2023 Jordan Parry
All rights reserved.

No portion of this book may be reproduced in any form without written permission from the publisher or author, except as permitted by U.S. copyright law.

This publication is designed to provide accurate and authoritative information in regard to the subject matter covered. It is sold with the understanding that neither the author nor the publisher is engaged in rendering legal, investment, accounting or other professional services. While the publisher and author have used their best efforts in preparing this book, they make no representations or warranties with respect to the accuracy or completeness of the contents of this book and specifically disclaim any implied warranties of merchantability or fitness for a particular purpose. No warranty may be created or extended by sales representatives or written sales materials. The advice and strategies contained herein may not be suitable for your situation. You should consult with a professional when appropriate. Neither the publisher nor the author shall be liable for any loss of profit or any other commercial damages, including but not limited to special, incidental, consequential, personal, or other damages.

Bonus!

Get this **FREE** book by signing up to our positivity club. Plus be the first to receive all my latest books completely FREE!

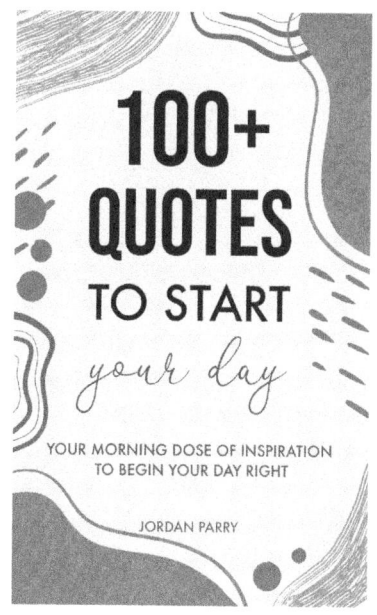

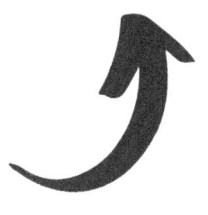

Scan this QR code with
your camera to sign up!

Table of contents

Introduction 7

Understanding Affirmations 9

Benefits for Expectant Mothers 11

Making Affirmations Work: Practical Tips and Techniques 15

Affirmations 19

Thank you! 111

Introduction

Pregnancy is not just a period of physical transformation, but also a profound journey of the heart and soul. As you nurture the life growing within you, you are also nurturing an evolving version of yourself, poised on the brink of a beautiful new chapter. "Blossoming Within: Affirmations for Expectant Mothers" has been lovingly crafted to accompany you on this extraordinary journey.

This book is a collection of empowering affirmations, aimed at emboldening you, soothing your worries, and celebrating the miraculous process that is pregnancy. Each affirmation is a seed, sown to grow into a powerful belief, a beacon of positivity that can light your path through the ups and downs of this transformative period.

The pages of this book are filled with affirmations designed to remind you of your inner strength, your body's remarkable capabilities, and the boundless love that already exists between you and your unborn child.Welcome to your journey of blossoming within.

Understanding Affirmations

As we embark on the journey of exploring affirmations, it's crucial to understand what they really are. At their core, affirmations are positive statements or declarations that are used to challenge and overcome self-sabotaging and negative thoughts. They are a powerful tool that can help you reshape your mindset and cultivate a more positive, empowering perspective towards various aspects of your life.

Affirmations are based on the principles of neuroplasticity, the brain's ability to reorganize itself by forming new neural connections. When we repeat a positive affirmation, we're essentially training our brain to believe this statement. Over time, our subconscious mind begins to accept this affirmation as a fundamental truth, thereby influencing our behaviors, habits, and attitudes in line with this new belief.

For instance, an affirmation like "I am strong and capable" not only boosts your self-confidence but also reinforces your belief in your ability to face and overcome challenges. When repeated consistently, this affirmation can foster resilience, equipping you to navigate life's ups and downs with greater strength and grace.

Pregnancy is a time of profound change, a period filled with excitement, anticipation, and often, a fair share of anxiety. Affirmations can be especially beneficial during this transformative phase. They can help you embrace the changes in your body, build a deep sense of connection with the life growing inside you, and prepare you emotionally for the journey of motherhood.

However, the power of affirmations extends beyond simply uttering positive words. The true essence of an affirmation lies in the emotion and belief behind it. As you recite an affirmation, it's important to visualize it, to feel it, and to genuinely believe in it. This emotional engagement can significantly amplify the impact of the affirmation, making it a potent force that can shape your reality.

Remember, every affirmation you choose to recite is a step towards creating a positive, nurturing environment for both you and your baby. Embrace them, believe in them, and let them guide you on this beautiful journey.

Benefits for Expectant Mothers

Pregnancy is a profound journey, one that brings with it a whirlwind of emotions and changes, both physical and emotional. Amidst this transformative period, affirmations can serve as a gentle, empowering guide, providing numerous benefits to expectant mothers. Let's delve into how these potent declarations can positively influence your pregnancy journey.

1. Cultivating Positive Emotions: One of the primary benefits of affirmations lies in their ability to foster positivity. When you repeat statements like, "I am filled with joy and gratitude for the life growing inside me," you're encouraging a more optimistic perspective. This not only enhances your overall well-being but also creates a serene emotional environment for your baby.

2. Boosting Self-confidence: Pregnancy, especially for first-time mothers, can sometimes bring feelings of uncertainty or inadequacy. Affirmations like, "I trust in my ability to birth my baby," can bolster your self-confidence, reminding you of your innate strength and resilience.

3.Reducing Stress and Anxiety: Pregnancy can be a time of heightened anxiety. Affirmations serve as a grounding force, helping to allay fears and worries. When coupled with deep breathing or meditation, affirmations like "I am calm, I am safe, my baby is safe," can promote relaxation and ease anxiety.

4.Strengthening the Mother-Baby Bond: Affirmations can also enhance the emotional connection between you and your unborn child. As you affirm, "I love my baby, and my baby feels my love," you're fostering a deep bond of love and trust, even before you've physically met your baby.

5.Preparing for Birth: The process of childbirth can seem daunting for many women. Affirmations can help to mentally and emotionally prepare you for this process. Statements like, "My body is designed to give birth efficiently and smoothly," can alleviate fears surrounding childbirth, instilling confidence in your body's natural capabilities.

6.Encouraging a Healthy Body Image: Pregnancy brings about significant changes to your body, which can sometimes lead to feelings of discomfort or self-consciousness. Affirmations like "I embrace the changes in my body with love and respect" can help promote a positive body image, aiding you in lovingly accepting your transforming body.

7.Promoting a Mindset of Acceptance and Surrender: Pregnancy is a time of change and uncertainty. Affirmations can help you cultivate a mindset of acceptance and surrender, enabling you to navigate this journey with grace and resilience.

Remember, the power of affirmations lies not just in the words, but in the belief behind them. As you journey through pregnancy, let these affirmations be your guide, your mantra, your source of strength. Embrace their positivity, feel their power, and let them illuminate your path to motherhood.

Making Affirmations Work: Practical Tips and Techniques

Harnessing the power of affirmations can profoundly transform your pregnancy journey, but it's essential to know how to use them effectively. Here, we'll discuss key points on how to incorporate affirmations into your daily life and maximize their impact.

1. Consistency is Key: Much like physical exercise, the benefits of affirmations are felt over time with regular practice. Make it a habit to say your affirmations daily. You might want to incorporate them into your morning routine or use them as a calming practice before bed.

2. Personalize Your Affirmations: While this book provides many affirmations for you, it can be powerful to create your own. Use positive, present tense language, and frame them in a way that resonates with your personal experiences and emotions. For example, "I am nurturing my baby with love and care every day."

3. Engage Emotionally: The effectiveness of affirmations lies not just in the words, but in the emotion and belief behind them. As you recite an affirmation, visualize it, feel it, and believe it.

This deep emotional engagement amplifies its power.

4.Combine with Relaxation Techniques: Pairing affirmations with relaxation techniques like deep breathing, meditation, or yoga can enhance their effectiveness. For instance, you could inhale deeply while thinking "I am calm," and exhale while thinking "I release all tension."

5.Use Affirmations throughout the Day: While having a dedicated time for affirmations is beneficial, using them throughout the day can reinforce their impact. Repeat them silently to yourself during routine activities, or when you're feeling stressed or anxious.

6.Write Them Down: Writing your affirmations down in a journal or on sticky notes placed around your home can help reinforce their message. Seeing these positive statements regularly reminds your brain of their truth, reinforcing the new neural pathways you're building.

7.Be Patient with Yourself: Change doesn't happen overnight. It may take time for an affirmation to feel true for you, and that's okay. Be patient with yourself, and remember, the journey is just as important as the destination.

8.Use the Notes Section: To help you personalize this journey, we've included a special section at the back of the book, designed for you to make your own notes. Remember to use this space to record your experiences, feelings, or any new affirmations you come up with. This will help you track your progress and make this journey more personalized.

With regular practice, these positive statements can become your natural thought patterns, providing a foundation of strength, positivity, and calm as you navigate the beautiful journey of pregnancy.

Affirmations

I am strong and capable of nurturing new life.

...

My body is a miracle, growing and protecting my baby.

...

I trust my body to know what to do throughout my pregnancy.

...

I am surrounded by love and support during this journey.

...

My baby and I are connected and bonded.

...

I deserve happiness, health, and love during my pregnancy.

I am grateful for the gift of creating new life.

...

I am patient and trust the process of pregnancy.

...

I am capable of handling any challenges that arise during pregnancy.

...

My baby is growing and developing beautifully.

...

I am a powerful and loving mother-to-be.

...

I am confident in my ability to give birth.

...

My body is wise and knows exactly how to care for my baby.

I embrace the changes in my body with love and gratitude.

...

I am worthy of a joyful and healthy pregnancy.

...

My baby feels my love and care.

...

I am prepared to make the best choices for my baby.

...

I am in tune with my body's needs and signals.

...

I am surrounded by positivity and love.

...

I cherish each moment of my pregnancy journey.

I am filled with joy and gratitude for the life growing inside me.

...

I am growing stronger and more resilient every day.

...

My baby and I are a team, working together towards a healthy birth.

...

I welcome the support of others during this special time.

...

My body is a safe and nurturing environment for my baby.

...

I trust in my instincts as a mother-to-be.

I am calm and at ease during my pregnancy.

...

I am grateful for my body's ability to grow and nourish my baby.

...

I am surrounded by a supportive community of family and friends.

...

I am flexible and adaptable during my pregnancy journey.

...

I am patient with myself and my body as it changes.

...

I am proud of the life I am creating.

I am capable of handling any emotions that arise during my pregnancy.

...

I believe in my ability to be an amazing mother.

...

I am prepared for the arrival of my baby.

...

I am strong and resilient in mind, body, and spirit.

...

I am a source of love and comfort for my baby.

...

I am excited for the journey ahead.

...

I am focused on a healthy and peaceful pregnancy.

I am at peace with the changes in my body.

...

I am a nurturing and loving mother-to-be.

...

I am gentle with myself during this transformative time.

...

My baby is growing strong and healthy inside me.

...

I am confident in my body's ability to birth my baby.

...

I am connected to my inner wisdom and intuition.

I am deserving of a beautiful birth experience.

...

My baby and I are thriving together.

...

I am grateful for the opportunity to bring new life into the world.

...

I am committed to a healthy and happy pregnancy.

...

I am prepared to nurture and care for my baby.

...

I am a loving and attentive mother-to-be.

...

My baby is a blessing and a gift.

I am embracing the changes in my body with grace and gratitude.

...

I am confident in my ability to make wise decisions for my baby.

...

I am a source of strength and love for my baby.

...

I am capable of overcoming any obstacles during my pregnancy.

...

I am committed to self-care and nurturing myself during this time.

...

I am grateful for the support and love of those around me.

I am strong and courageous as a mother-to-be.

...

I am focused on my and my baby's well-being.

...

I am giving my baby the best possible start in life.

...

I am grateful for the strength and resilience of my body.

...

I am in tune with my body's natural rhythms and signals.

...

I am filled with love and positivity during my pregnancy.

I am confident in my body's ability to heal and nourish itself.

...

I am deserving of all the love and support I receive.

...

I am calm, I am safe, my baby is safe.

...

I am a powerful and courageous mother-to-be.

...

I am connected to my baby on a deep and spiritual level.

...

I am embracing this journey with an open heart and mind.

I am grateful for the wisdom and guidance of my healthcare providers.

...

I am a loving and nurturing presence for my baby.

...

I am in control of my thoughts and emotions during pregnancy.

...

I am at peace with the physical and emotional changes I experience.

...

I am focused on creating a peaceful and loving environment for my baby.

...

I am dedicated to nurturing my baby's growth and development.

I trust in my ability to birth my baby.

...

I am confident in my ability to provide for my baby's needs.

...

I am grateful for the unique and beautiful experience of pregnancy.

...

I am constantly learning and growing as a mother-to-be.

...

I am gentle with myself and my body during this time of change.

...

I am creating a loving and secure bond with my baby.

I am surrounded by people who care for and support me.

...

I am open to the guidance and wisdom of others.

...

I am filled with a deep sense of purpose and joy as a mother-to-be.

...

I am committed to maintaining a healthy lifestyle for my baby and me.

...

I am deserving of all the beauty and joy that motherhood brings.

...

I am confident in my ability to make the best choices for my baby.

I am embracing my new role as a mother with love and enthusiasm.

...

I am open to receiving help and support from those around me.

...

I am filled with love and gratitude for my growing baby.

...

I am confident in my ability to navigate the challenges of pregnancy.

...

I am focused on creating a positive and nurturing environment for my baby.

...

I am connected to a network of strong and supportive mothers.

I am a source of unconditional love for my baby.

...

I am patient with myself as I adjust to the changes in my body and life.

...

I am secure in my role as a mother-to-be.

...

I am open to the lessons and growth that pregnancy offers.

...

I am excited to share my love and care with my baby.

...

I am dedicated to being the best mother I can be.

I am nurturing a healthy and loving connection with my baby.

...

I am grateful for each day of my pregnancy journey.

...

I am a powerful, loving, and confident mother-to-be.

...

I am embracing the beautiful journey of motherhood with grace and courage.

...

I am learning to trust my intuition as a mother-to-be.

...

I am grateful for the opportunity to love and nurture my baby.

I am prioritizing self-care to ensure my well-being during pregnancy.

...

I am growing and evolving alongside my baby.

...

I am taking time to connect with my baby each day.

...

I am focused on creating beautiful memories during my pregnancy.

...

I am a beacon of love and support for my baby.

...

I am filled with excitement and anticipation for my baby's arrival.

I am constantly surrounded by positive energy and love.

...

I am grateful for the ability to provide a loving home for my baby.

...

I am confident in my ability to balance my needs and my baby's needs.

...

I am in awe of the incredible journey my body is going through.

...

I am surrounded by a circle of love and support from family and friends.

...

I am a strong and capable mother, ready to face any challenges.

I am experiencing the beauty and miracle of pregnancy every day.

...

I am finding joy and wonder in the small moments of my pregnancy.

...

I am embracing the transformation that motherhood brings.

...

I am giving myself permission to rest and recharge during my pregnancy.

...

I am honoring the incredible power of my body to create and sustain life.

...

I am releasing any fears and anxieties related to pregnancy and birth.

I am trusting that the universe has a beautiful plan for me and my baby.

...

I am cultivating a deep sense of inner peace and calm during my pregnancy.

...

I am a loving and compassionate mother-to-be.

...

I am a source of strength and inspiration for my baby.

...

I am creating a healthy and supportive environment for my growing baby.

...

I am nurturing my body with love, care, and nourishment.

I am a powerful force of love and light during my pregnancy.

...

I am celebrating the miracle of life within me.

...

I am honoring and cherishing the sacred bond between my baby and me.

...

I am committed to being present and engaged in each moment of my pregnancy.

...

I am confident in my ability to navigate the transitions of motherhood.

...

I am embracing my body's wisdom and abilities during pregnancy.

I am cultivating a loving and joyful connection with my baby.

...

I am filled with gratitude and awe for the gift of motherhood.

...

I am open to the wisdom and guidance of other mothers.

...

I am celebrating the unique and incredible journey of my pregnancy.

...

I am honoring my body's strength and resilience during pregnancy.

...

I am focused on creating a safe and loving space for my baby to grow.

I am a loving, capable, and devoted mother-to-be.

...

I am finding balance and harmony during my pregnancy journey.

...

I am growing and evolving as a mother every day.

...

I am connecting with my baby through love, care, and communication.

...

I am prepared for the joys and challenges of motherhood.

...

I am prioritizing my mental, emotional, and physical well-being during pregnancy.

I am feeling more confident and capable as a mother-to-be each day.

...

I am embracing the power and beauty of my pregnant body.

...

I am cultivating patience and understanding during my pregnancy.

...

I am filled with a sense of wonder and excitement for my baby's arrival.

...

I am committed to creating a loving and nurturing home for my baby.

...

I am honoring the sacred journey of motherhood with gratitude and reverence.

I am finding joy and fulfillment in the process of becoming a mother.

...

I am embracing the changes in my body with love and acceptance.

...

I am nourishing my body, mind, and spirit during pregnancy.

...

I am learning to trust the natural instincts that guide me as a mother.

...

I am a source of calm and tranquility for my baby.

...

I am celebrating the unique gifts and qualities that I bring as a mother.

I am embracing the incredible bond between my baby and me.

...

I am taking time to cherish and appreciate the miracle of pregnancy.

...

I am discovering the depths of my love and devotion as a mother-to-be.

...

I am cultivating inner strength and resilience during my pregnancy journey.

...

I am grateful for the loving support of my partner, family, and friends.

...

I am nurturing a deep sense of self-love and self-compassion during pregnancy.

I am confident in my ability to make the best choices for my baby and me.

...

I am focusing on the beauty and joy of my pregnancy journey.

...

I am creating a strong foundation of love and support for my baby.

...

I am mindful of the incredible power and responsibility of motherhood.

...

I am embracing the growth and learning that pregnancy brings.

...

I am honoring the beauty of my pregnant body in all its forms.

I am a loving and caring presence for my baby throughout my pregnancy.

...

I am embracing the wisdom and guidance of my healthcare providers.

...

I am cultivating a sense of calm and serenity during my pregnancy.

...

I am excited and prepared for the adventure of motherhood.

...

I am finding strength and support in the community of mothers around me.

...

I am a courageous and resilient mother-to-be, ready for the journey ahead.

I am focused on the well-being of my baby and myself during pregnancy.

...

I am developing a deeper connection with my baby each day.

...

I am committed to self-care and self-compassion during this transformative time.

...

I am appreciating the gift of life that I am carrying within me.

...

I am growing in wisdom and understanding as a mother-to-be.

...

I am cherishing the opportunity to bond with my baby before birth.

I am trusting my body's innate ability to nurture and protect my baby.

...

I am embracing the natural rhythms and cycles of pregnancy.

...

I am celebrating the love and joy that my baby brings into my life.

...

I am grateful for the ability to experience the miracle of motherhood.

...

I am learning to be patient and gentle with myself during pregnancy.

...

I am cultivating a deep sense of gratitude for the journey of motherhood.

I am honoring my body's incredible ability to create and sustain life.

...

I am nurturing my baby with love, care, and positive energy.

...

I am welcoming the new experiences and challenges of motherhood with open arms.

...

I am discovering new depths of love and connection with my baby.

...

I am committed to being a loving and supportive presence for my baby.

...

I am embracing the unique and beautiful journey of pregnancy and motherhood.

I am finding strength and courage within myself as a mother-to-be.

...

I am honoring the sacred and profound experience of carrying new life.

...

I am celebrating the transformation and growth that pregnancy brings.

...

I am cultivating a loving and nurturing environment for my baby to thrive.

...

I am connecting with my baby on a deep and meaningful level.

...

I am focused on the present moment, cherishing each day of my pregnancy journey.

I am a confident, loving, and capable mother-to-be, ready to embrace the adventure of motherhood.

...

I am embracing each stage of pregnancy as a unique and precious moment.

...

I am choosing to fill my mind with positive and empowering thoughts.

...

I am learning to trust and respect my body's natural wisdom and capabilities.

...

I am choosing to nourish my body with foods that promote my well-being and my baby's development.

I am connected to a powerful lineage of mothers and motherhood.

...

I am lovingly preparing for the arrival of my baby.

...

I am experiencing the beauty and wonder of creating life every day.

...

I am consciously creating peaceful and joyful experiences for me and my baby.

...

I am filled with radiant health and vitality during my pregnancy.

...

I am creating a sacred space within me for my baby to grow and develop.

I am approaching my due date with excitement and serenity.

...

I am ready to welcome my baby into a world filled with love and positivity.

...

I am expressing my needs and feelings openly and honestly during my pregnancy.

...

I am treating myself with kindness and patience as I navigate the journey of pregnancy.

...

I am embracing the shifts in my lifestyle as a part of the journey to motherhood.

...

I am allowing myself to feel all emotions fully, without judgment.

I am confident in my body's ability to move through labor and birth.

...

I am consciously sending love and light to my baby every day.

...

I am creating a birth plan that honors my needs and preferences.

...

I am trusting the journey, knowing that every step brings me closer to meeting my baby.

...

I am empowering myself with knowledge about pregnancy, birth, and motherhood.

...

I am allowing my intuition to guide my decisions during pregnancy and childbirth.

I am cherishing the quiet moments of connection with my baby.

...

I am giving myself permission to ask for help and support when I need it.

...

I am welcoming the changes in my body as signs of my baby's growth and development.

...

I am mindfully embracing the transformation that pregnancy brings to my body, mind, and spirit.

...

I am confident that I will be an excellent role model for my child.

...

I am committed to maintaining balance in all aspects of my life during pregnancy.

I am ready to experience the joy and challenge of breastfeeding my baby.

...

I am aware of my body's strength and potential to birth my baby naturally.

...

I am celebrating the anticipation and excitement that each new day of pregnancy brings.

...

I am listening to my body's needs and taking rest when required.

...

I am creating a peaceful and harmonious environment for my baby to come home to.

...

I am welcoming each new experience during pregnancy as an opportunity for growth.

I am taking time to envision the loving relationship I will have with my baby.

...

I am choosing to fill my heart with hope and anticipation for my baby's arrival.

...

I am committed to maintaining a positive and optimistic outlook during my pregnancy.

...

I am confident in my ability to handle the transition to motherhood with grace.

...

I am fostering a strong bond with my baby through my thoughts and emotions.

...

I am a beautiful and radiant mother-to-be.

I am surrounded by an aura of protection and love during my pregnancy.

...

I am looking forward to the journey of discovering my baby's unique personality.

...

I am resilient and flexible, adapting to the changes that pregnancy brings.

...

I am honoring my body's need for rest and rejuvenation during pregnancy.

...

I am nurturing my mind with positive thoughts and empowering beliefs.

...

I am prepared to meet any challenges during my pregnancy with courage and grace.

I am ready to embark on the amazing journey of parenthood.

...

I am experiencing the profound bond between a mother and her unborn child.

...

I am embracing every moment of my pregnancy as a gift and a blessing.

...

I am letting go of any fears or anxieties about childbirth.

...

I am finding joy and contentment in my journey to motherhood.

...

I am ready to embrace the changes that motherhood will bring to my life.

I am prepared to welcome the changes in my body with love and acceptance.

...

I am looking forward to sharing my love with my little one.

...

I am aware that my positive thoughts are influencing my baby's development.

...

I am creating a safe and secure world for my baby.

...

I am committed to taking care of my health and well-being during pregnancy.

...

I am accepting the unique journey of my pregnancy with gratitude and openness.

I am ready to love and care for my baby with all my heart.

...

I am patiently awaiting the arrival of my baby with joy and anticipation.

...

I am finding strength in the love and support of my family and friends.

...

I am excited to share the journey of motherhood with my partner.

...

I am embracing the wisdom and intuition that come with pregnancy.

...

I am creating an environment of peace and harmony for my baby.

I am accepting all the emotions that come with pregnancy without judgement.

...

I am taking care of my physical health to ensure a healthy pregnancy.

...

I am filled with a sense of wonder and amazement at the life growing inside me.

...

I am prepared to embrace the changes and challenges that come with motherhood.

...

I am ready to share my life and my love with my baby.

...

I am confident that my baby feels my love and care.

I am nurturing my spirit and mind, preparing for the journey of motherhood.

...

I am patient with myself, understanding that every stage of pregnancy is unique.

...

I am ready to adapt to the new routines and rhythms that come with motherhood.

...

I am cherishing the intimate bond I am forming with my baby.

...

I am a beacon of love and positivity for my baby.

...

I am aware of my body's innate wisdom and strength during pregnancy.

I am fully present in each moment, cherishing the journey of pregnancy.

...

I am eagerly anticipating the joy of holding my baby in my arms.

...

I am grateful for the opportunity to experience the miracle of childbirth.

...

I am a strong and capable woman, ready to become a mother.

...

I am accepting and appreciating the changes in my body with love.

...

I am blessed with the gift of creating and nurturing life.

I am calmly preparing my mind and body for a healthy childbirth.

...

I am creating a strong bond with my baby, even before birth.

...

I am deeply connected to the life force within me.

...

I am embracing every change as a sign of a healthy pregnancy.

...

I am confident in my ability to provide a safe and loving environment for my baby.

...

I am finding peace and comfort in the rhythm of my baby's movements.

I am gracefully transitioning into the role of a mother.

...

I am hopeful and excited about the future with my baby.

...

I am in tune with my body's natural rhythms and cycles.

...

I am joyful and content in every stage of my pregnancy.

...

I am kind and gentle with myself as I navigate this new journey.

...

I am lovingly preparing my body and mind for the arrival of my baby.

I am nourishing my body with wholesome foods that support my baby's growth.

...

I am open to the wonders and miracles of pregnancy.

...

I am patient, knowing that my body is doing exactly what it needs to for my baby.

...

I am quietly communicating my love and care to my baby.

...

I am radiating positive energy and joy during my pregnancy.

...

I am treasuring each moment and movement as my baby grows.

I am unconditionally loving my body as it nurtures new life.

...

I am visualizing a safe and healthy birth for my baby.

...

I am welcoming the new experiences and growth that come with motherhood.

...

I am excited to embark on this new chapter of my life.

...

I am nourishing my baby with my thoughts, feelings, and physical well-being.

...

My body is designed to give birth efficiently and smoothly.

I am ready to love, cherish, and care for my baby.

...

I am surrounded by positivity and love during my pregnancy.

...

I am trusting my instincts and intuition to guide me through my pregnancy.

...

I am valuing each day of my pregnancy as a day closer to meeting my baby.

...

I am welcoming the joy and love that my baby brings into my life.

...

I am experiencing the joy and beauty of pregnancy every day.

I am focused on creating a loving and nurturing environment for my baby.

...

I am growing and changing in the best ways for my baby.

...

I am honoring the incredible journey my body is going through.

...

I am joyfully anticipating the arrival of my baby.

...

I am listening to my body's needs and responding with love and care.

...

I am nourishing my baby with every breath I take.

I am opening my heart to the endless love I have for my baby.

...

I am prepared to meet my baby with love, patience, and joy.

...

I am ready to provide everything my baby needs to grow and thrive.

...

I am strengthening my mind and body for childbirth.

...

I am taking time to rest and rejuvenate, for myself and my baby.

...

I am understanding that every moment of pregnancy is a moment of creation.

I am visualizing a healthy and happy baby growing inside me.

...

I am welcoming the transformation that motherhood brings.

...

I am embracing the beauty and power of my pregnant body.

...

I am confident in my ability to birth my baby.

...

I am nourishing my body and my baby with healthy and nutritious food.

...

I am relaxed and at peace, knowing that childbirth is a natural process.

I am grounded and centered in the experience of my pregnancy.

...

I am embracing the love and excitement that each day brings closer to my baby's arrival.

...

I am fostering an environment of peace and positivity for my baby.

...

I am grateful for the miracle of life growing inside me.

...

I am honoring my body's wisdom and power in creating new life.

...

I am joyful in anticipation of the day I will hold my baby in my arms.

I am kind to my body, giving it the rest and care it needs during this time.

...

I am lovingly preparing myself for the journey of motherhood.

...

I am mindful of the precious gift of life within me.

...

I am nurturing a deep connection with my baby.

...

I am open to all the possibilities that motherhood will bring.

...

I am positive that I am doing the best for my baby and me.

I am resting when I need to, knowing that it is beneficial for my baby and me.

...

I am soothed by the rhythm of my baby's heartbeat.

...

I am thankful for the love and support I am receiving during my pregnancy.

...

I am understanding of my body's needs during this transformative time.

...

I am visualizing a smooth and safe delivery.

...

I am welcoming the journey to motherhood with an open heart.

I am excited about the new beginnings that my baby brings.

...

I am grateful for the strength and resilience of my body.

...

I am healing and recovering in preparation for the arrival of my baby.

...

I am intuitively making the best decisions for my baby and me.

...

I am joyful and radiant, embracing the changes in my body.

...

I am kind to myself, acknowledging the incredible work my body is doing.

I am lovingly communicating with my baby every day.

...

I am mindful of the importance of balance during my pregnancy.

...

I am nurturing my body with the right exercises during my pregnancy.

...

I am optimistic about the wonderful journey of motherhood ahead.

...

I am proud of the amazing work my body is doing to create a new life.

...

I am ready for the profound joy and love that comes with holding my baby.

I am strong and prepared for the journey of childbirth.

...

I am thankful for every day that brings me closer to meeting my baby.

...

I am understanding that every woman's pregnancy journey is unique and special.

...

I am visualizing my baby growing healthy and strong.

...

I am welcoming each new day with joy and anticipation.

...

I am excited for the special bond I will share with my baby.

I am growing a healthy, happy baby inside me.

...

I am honoring the special time of pregnancy as a time of transformation.

...

I am joyful in the knowledge that I am creating a new life.

...

I am kind and patient with myself during this time of change.

...

I am loving the feeling of my baby moving inside me.

...

I am mindful of my thoughts and feelings, knowing they affect my baby.

I am nurturing my soul with positive thoughts and peaceful moments.

...

I am open to the changes and adaptations my body is making.

...

I am patient and calm as I await the arrival of my baby.

...

I am resilient, strong, and ready to become a mother.

...

I am thankful for the life I am creating.

...

I am understanding and patient with the changes in my body.

I love my baby, and my baby feels my love.

...

I am visualizing a peaceful and joyous birth.

...

I am welcoming the sacred journey of motherhood.

...

I am excited to witness the miracle of birth.

...

I am growing stronger and more resilient each day.

...

I am honoring my body's signals and taking care of my health.

I am joyful in the anticipation of the new life I am bringing into the world.

...

I am kind and loving to myself as I navigate this transformative journey.

...

I am loving the deepening connection between my baby and me.

...

I am mindful of my nutrition, knowing it directly affects my baby's health.

...

I am nurturing a sense of peace and calm within myself for my baby.

...

I am open to receiving help and support from others during my pregnancy.

I am patient, knowing that each day brings me closer to meeting my baby.

...

I am resilient in facing any challenges that come my way.

...

I am thankful for the remarkable journey that pregnancy is.

...

I am understanding of my emotions and allow myself to feel them fully.

...

I am visualizing my body confidently carrying and birthing my baby.

...

I am welcoming the changes that are making me a mother.

I am excited for the endless love I will share with my baby.

...

I am growing as a person as I prepare to become a mother.

...

I am honoring this special time in my life and taking time to rest and rejuvenate.

...

I am joyful and vibrant, radiating positivity for my baby.

...

I am kind to my body, acknowledging the hard work it is doing.

...

I am loving the unique journey that each day of pregnancy brings.

I am mindful of the strength and power within me.

...

I am nurturing my body with healthy habits and routines.

...

I am open to the lessons that motherhood will teach me.

...

I am patient with the process and trust my body's wisdom.

...

I am resilient and capable, ready for the journey of motherhood.

...

I am thankful for the miracle of life I am experiencing.

I am understanding of my body's changes and embrace them with love.

...

I am visualizing a healthy and happy baby.

...

I am welcoming the new experiences that motherhood will bring.

...

I am excited to share my world with my little one.

...

I am growing a strong and healthy baby inside me.

...

I am honoring my pregnancy as a time of beauty and transformation.

I am joyful, knowing I will soon meet my baby.

...

I am kind, understanding, and patient with myself during this journey.

...

I am loving my body for the amazing work it is doing.

...

I am mindful of my baby's movements and respond with love.

...

I am nurturing my mind with positive thoughts for me and my baby.

...

I am open to the beauty and mystery of childbirth.

I am patient with myself and my body as we prepare for birth.

...

I am resilient, knowing I have the strength to birth my baby.

...

I am thankful for each day that brings me closer to holding my baby.

...

I am understanding of my body's needs and prioritize self-care.

...

I am visualizing a smooth and peaceful birthing process.

...

I am welcoming my baby with a heart full of love and joy.

I am excited to embrace all aspects of motherhood.

...

I am growing into a role that I was destined for – being a mother.

...

I am honoring the changes in my body as signs of its strength and capability.

...

I am joyful in knowing I will soon hold my baby in my arms.

...

I am kind to myself, taking each day of pregnancy as it comes.

...

I am loving the journey of pregnancy, with all its ups and downs.

I am mindful of my well-being, knowing it influences my baby's health.

...

I am nurturing my body and mind with rest and relaxation.

...

I am open to learning new things about myself and my baby each day.

...

I am patient and understanding, knowing that every phase of pregnancy is important.

...

I am resilient in the face of any challenges that come my way.

...

I am thankful for the unique experience of carrying and nurturing life.

I am understanding of my body's needs and respond with care.

...

I am visualizing the moment when I will finally meet my baby.

...

I am welcoming the growth and transformation that pregnancy brings.

...

I am excited to feel the powerful love that comes with motherhood.

...

I am growing a bond with my baby that will last a lifetime.

...

I am honoring myself as a woman capable of creating and nurturing life.

I am joyful, celebrating the life that is growing inside me.

...

I am kind to my body, treating it with love and respect.

...

I am loving every moment that brings me closer to meeting my baby.

...

I am mindful of my mental health, knowing it's important for my baby and me.

...

I am nurturing my spirit with thoughts of love, peace, and joy.

...

I am open to the natural process of birth.

I am patient, knowing that my body is working perfectly in its own time.

...

I am resilient, empowered by the journey of pregnancy.

...

I am thankful for the opportunity to become a mother.

...

I am understanding of the emotions that come with pregnancy.

...

I am visualizing a healthy and happy life for my baby.

...

I am welcoming my baby into a world full of love and care.

I am excited to share my life's journey with my little one.

...

I am growing stronger and more capable each day.

...

I am honoring the miracle of life that is unfolding within me.

...

I am joyful, radiating positivity to my baby.

...

I am kind and gentle with myself as I navigate pregnancy.

...

I am loving the connection that is growing between my baby and me.

I am mindful of the needs of my body and baby.

...

I am nurturing my baby with every heartbeat.

...

I am open to the wisdom that pregnancy and motherhood bring.

...

I am patient, understanding that good things take time.

...

I am resilient, knowing that I have everything I need within me.

...

I am thankful for this special time in my life.

I am understanding of the changes happening in my body.

...

I am visualizing a peaceful and joyous birthing experience.

...

I am welcoming the blessings that my baby brings.

...

I am excited about the memories I will create with my baby.

...

I am growing a healthy baby with each passing day.

...

I am honoring my journey to motherhood.

I am joyful, embracing the journey of pregnancy.

...

I am kind to myself, understanding that rest is important.

...

I am loving the new experiences that pregnancy brings.

...

I am nurturing my body, mind, and spirit for the arrival of my baby.

...

I am open to the love and happiness my baby will bring into my life.

...

I am patient with the process and trust in the timing of my body.

I am resilient, prepared for the journey of childbirth and motherhood.

...

I am thankful for each kick, each movement I feel from my baby.

...

I am understanding of the needs of my body during pregnancy.

...

I am visualizing a positive birthing experience.

...

I am welcoming the joy that comes with the anticipation of my baby's arrival.

...

I am excited to see my baby grow and develop.

I am growing emotionally stronger each day of my pregnancy.

...

I am honoring my body's incredible ability to create life.

...

I am joyful, knowing that my baby will soon be in my arms.

...

I am kind and loving to myself and my growing baby.

...

I am loving the anticipation of meeting my baby.

...

I am mindful of my baby's presence, cherishing each movement.

I am nurturing a deep and powerful bond with my baby.

...

I am open to the new and exciting journey of motherhood.

...

I am patient, knowing that each day brings me closer to my baby.

...

I am resilient, facing each day of pregnancy with strength and grace.

...

I am thankful for the amazing journey of becoming a mother.

...

I am understanding of my body's changes and embrace them with positivity.

I am visualizing my baby healthy, happy, and thriving.

...

I am welcoming my baby into my life with endless love and joy.

...

I am excited to share my love and wisdom with my child.

...

I am growing into the best version of myself for my baby.

...

I am honoring each day of my pregnancy as a miracle.

...

I am joyful in anticipation of the wonderful times ahead.

I am kind to myself, nourishing my body with care and respect.

...

I am loving every moment I spend connecting with my baby.

...

I am mindful of the incredible journey that motherhood will be.

...

I am nurturing my body and soul, preparing for the birth of my baby.

...

I am open to the incredible changes that motherhood will bring.

...

I am patient, knowing my baby is developing at the perfect pace.

I am resilient, embracing the challenges of pregnancy with courage.

...

I am thankful for this precious time of anticipation and preparation.

...

I am understanding of my emotional journey during pregnancy.

...

I am visualizing my baby's safe and smooth arrival into the world.

...

I am welcoming the transformative journey of motherhood with open arms.

NOTES

NOTES

NOTES

NOTES

NOTES

Bonus!

Get this **FREE** book by signing up to our positivity club. Plus be the first to receive all my latest books completely FREE!

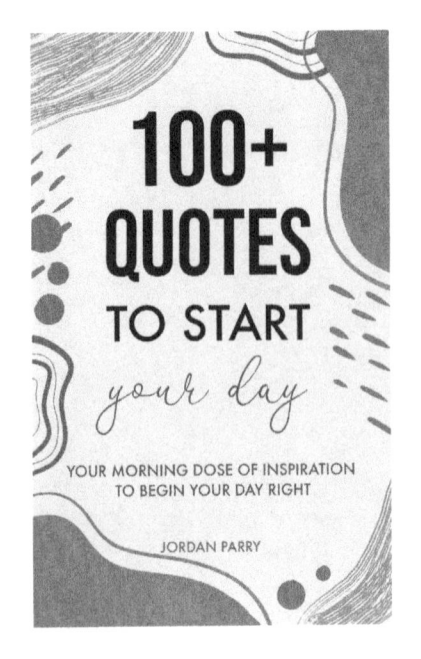

Scan this QR code with
your camera to sign up!

Thank you!

Thank you for choosing to read this book. We hope that this collection of powerful affirmations has provided you with valuable insights, inspiration, and motivation.

If you enjoyed the book, we would greatly appreciate it if you could take a moment to leave a review. Your feedback and insights are invaluable to us and help us to improve our work and provide better value to our readers.

In addition, we would like to invite you to visit our page where you can find out about our latest projects, download freebies and join our community of likeminded people. Let's learn, grow, and succeed together.

All our love,
Positive Change Press

www.positivechangepress.com

Made in the USA
Monee, IL
11 June 2024